Estrogen Diet for Women Over 40

A Beginner's Plan to Support Hormonal Balance Through Food, Sleep, and Lifestyle

mf

copyright © 2025 Mary Golanna

All rights reserved No part of this book may be reproduced, or stored in a retrieval system, or transmitted in any form or by any means, electronic, mechanical, photocopying, recording, or otherwise, without express written permission of the publisher.

Disclaimer

By reading this disclaimer, you are accepting the terms of the disclaimer in full. If you disagree with this disclaimer, please do not read the guide.

All of the content within this guide is provided for informational and educational purposes only, and should not be accepted as independent medical or other professional advice. The author is not a doctor, physician, nurse, mental health provider, or registered nutritionist/dietician. Therefore, using and reading this guide does not establish any form of a physician-patient relationship.

Always consult with a physician or another qualified health provider with any issues or questions you might have regarding any sort of medical condition. Do not ever disregard any qualified professional medical advice or delay seeking that advice because of anything you have read in this guide. The information in this guide is not intended to be any sort of medical advice and should not be used in lieu of any medical advice by a licensed and qualified medical professional.

The information in this guide has been compiled from a variety of known sources. However, the author cannot attest to or guarantee the accuracy of each source and thus should not be held liable for any errors or omissions.

You acknowledge that the publisher of this guide will not be held liable for any loss or damage of any kind incurred as a result of this guide or the reliance on any information provided within this guide. You acknowledge and agree that you assume all risk and responsibility for any action you undertake in response to the information in this guide.

Using this guide does not guarantee any particular result (e.g., weight loss or a cure). By reading this guide, you acknowledge that there are no guarantees to any specific outcome or results you can expect.

All product names, diet plans, or names used in this guide are for identification purposes only and are the property of their respective owners. The use of these names does not imply endorsement. All other trademarks cited herein are the property of their respective owners.

Where applicable, this guide is not intended to be a substitute for the original work of this diet plan and is, at most, a supplement to the original work for this diet plan and never a direct substitute. This guide is a personal expression of the facts of that diet plan.

Where applicable, persons shown in the cover images are stock photography models and the publisher has obtained the rights to use the images through license agreements with third-party stock image companies.

Table of Contents

Introduction — 7
Understanding Estrogen and Aging — 9
   What is Estrogen and Why is It Important? — 9
   What Happens to Hormones After 40 — 11
   Signs of Estrogen Imbalance — 13
   Estrogen Dominance vs. Estrogen Deficiency — 15
How Food Affects Hormones After 40 — 18
   Key Ways Food Impacts Hormones: — 18
   Estrogen-Supportive Nutrients — 19
   Foods that Help vs. Foods that Harm — 22
   The Role of Gut Health in Hormone Balance — 23
The Lifestyle Factors that Impact Estrogen — 25
   Sleep, Stress, and Cortisol — 25
   Exercise that Supports Hormonal Health — 27
   Environmental Toxins and Estrogen Disruptors — 29
Planning Your Hormone-Smart Kitchen — 33
   Pantry Essentials and Grocery List — 33
   How to Meal Prep with Hormones in Mind — 37
   Reading Labels and Avoiding Hidden Estrogen Disruptors — 40
Your 3-Week Estrogen Diet Plan — 42
   Week 1: Clean Out, Calm Down, Reset — 42
   Week 2: Nourish and Balance — 50
   Week 3: Thrive and Sustain — 56
Simple Recipes for Hormone Harmony — 63
   Breakfasts — 64
   Berry & Chia Hormone-Balancing Smoothie — 64
   Spinach & Mushroom Omelet — 65
   Flaxseed & Nut Butter Bowl — 66
   Avocado Toast With Sesame Seeds — 67

Phytoestrogen Smoothie Bowl	68
Lunches	69
Quinoa & Roasted Veggie Bowl	69
Hormone-Friendly Lentil Salad	70
Tofu Collard Wrap	71
Mediterranean Chickpea Bowl	72
Sweet Potato & Spinach Wrap	73
Dinners	74
Tofu Stir-Fry With Brown Rice	75
Roasted Chicken With Root Vegetables	76
Lentil & Spinach One-Pot Dish	77
Edamame Noodle Bowl	78
Snacks & Herbal Support	79
Sesame & Nut Energy Balls	79
Cucumber & Hummus Platter	80
Dark Chocolate & Walnut Toss	81
Chamomile & Lemon Tea	82
Apple & Almond Butter Snack	83
Sleep, Stress & Self-Care Essentials	**84**
Evening Wind-Down Routines	84
Natural Sleep Enhancers	86
Reducing Cortisol Through Breath, Boundaries, and Balance	87
Beyond the Diet: Long-Term Strategies for Hormonal Wellness	**89**
Supplements to Consider After 40	89
Tracking Symptoms and Progress	91
Staying Consistent Without Being Perfect	93
Conclusion	**96**
FAQs	**99**
References and Helpful Links	**102**

Introduction

Hormones are like the body's internal orchestra, each one playing a critical role in ensuring harmony and balance. But as you approach your 40s, that once-perfect symphony might start to feel a little off. Maybe you've noticed subtle shifts in your energy levels, sleep patterns, or the way your body responds to stress. Perhaps mood swings, stubborn weight gain, or irregular periods have made you wonder, "What's going on with my body?" If this sounds familiar, know this is a shared experience for many women.

After 40, your body undergoes a natural evolution, with hormone production changing in new ways. These shifts are part of a broader journey that includes perimenopause, menopause, and stepping into a new phase of life. While these changes are unavoidable, you have the power to navigate them. Through thoughtful food choices, lifestyle habits, and self-care, you can stay strong, vibrant, and in control of your body's story.

In this guide, we will talk about the following:

- Understanding Estrogen and Aging

- How Food Affects Hormones After 40
- The Lifestyle Factors That Impact Estrogen
- Planning Your Hormone-Smart Kitchen
- Your 3-Week Estrogen Diet Plan
- Simple Recipes for Hormone Harmony
- Beyond the Diet: Long-Term Strategies for Hormonal Wellness

Keep reading to learn more about how you can support your body through this transition and embrace the beauty of aging. By the end of this guide, you will have a better understanding of the physical, emotional, and mental changes that occur during menopause and how to manage them with grace and confidence.

Understanding Estrogen and Aging

Understanding the role of estrogen in our bodies is crucial when it comes to understanding menopause and aging. Estrogen, a hormone primarily produced by the ovaries, plays a significant role in reproductive health and bone strength.

It also affects other aspects of our health, such as cardiovascular health, brain function, skin elasticity, and muscle strength. This chapter will delve deeper into the functions of estrogen and how its levels change during menopause.

What is Estrogen and Why is It Important?

Estrogen is often referred to as the "*queen hormone*" because of its extensive impact on the female body. This hormone isn't just about reproduction; it governs a wide range of systems, including bone health, heart health, brain function, and even how your skin looks and feels. Estrogen acts like a manager, keeping the body's systems running smoothly.

For example, your brain relies on estrogen to regulate mood and cognitive sharpness. It also plays a role in maintaining joint flexibility, supporting a healthy gut lining, and even influencing how energy is stored or burned in the body. When levels are steady, you feel aligned and in sync. When estrogen is low or out of balance, those functions are compromised.

What Causes Estrogen Levels to Shift After 40?

Estrogen changes occur as part of the natural aging process. However, other factors, like chronic stress, diet, or exposure to environmental toxins, can speed up these changes or magnify their effects.

- *Perimenopause*: This can start as early as your mid-30s or as late as your mid-40s. During this phase, estrogen production begins to fluctuate, sometimes spiking and sometimes dipping.
- *Menopause*: This officially begins when you've gone 12 consecutive months without a menstrual period. At this stage, ovarian production of estrogen declines dramatically. The body becomes more reliant on fat tissue and adrenal glands to produce small amounts of estrogen.

These natural phases bring challenges, but they are also an opportunity to make intentional changes that nurture long-term wellness.

What Happens to Hormones After 40

Hormone changes start subtly as early as your late 30s, but the shifts are more noticeable in your 40s. Here's a breakdown of the most common hormonal trends at this age and how they affect your body and mind:

1. **Fluctuating Estrogen Levels**

   During perimenopause, estrogen levels can be unpredictable. Some months may be high, causing symptoms like breast tenderness or mood swings, while other months may see a sharp decline, leading to hot flashes or vaginal dryness. These swings can feel like an emotional rollercoaster, with days where you feel amazing followed by a sudden crash.

2. **Declining Progesterone**

   Progesterone, which balances estrogen, begins to decline faster than estrogen as you age. This often creates a hormonal imbalance called estrogen dominance, even if estrogen levels themselves are lower than they were in your 20s. Low progesterone often leads to disrupted sleep, anxiety, and heavy or irregular periods.

   Example: If you've noticed worsening PMS symptoms or difficulty sleeping despite being otherwise healthy, low progesterone could be the culprit.

3. **Reduced Testosterone**

   While testosterone is more commonly associated with men, women naturally produce a moderate amount of it, and it's essential for maintaining muscle mass, energy, and libido. Around 40, testosterone levels decline, which can lead to lower motivation, weaker muscles, and decreased sexual desire.

4. **Elevated Cortisol Levels**

   With age, your body becomes less resilient to stress. Chronic stress from a busy life, poor sleep, or nutrient deficiencies raises cortisol, the stress hormone. Elevated cortisol not only disrupts sleep and mood but also inhibits the body's ability to produce progesterone and estrogen.

5. **Insulin Sensitivity Wanes**

   Your body becomes less efficient at managing blood sugar as you age, which can lead to insulin resistance. Spikes and crashes in blood sugar impact hormones like cortisol and even estrogen. Eating a diet high in refined carbs or sugary snacks only worsens this cycle.

Taking gradual steps to manage these shifts with targeted nutrition, exercise, and self-care can make a tremendous difference over time.

Signs of Estrogen Imbalance

Hormonal imbalance doesn't happen overnight, and the symptoms are often varied. You might experience just one or two signs of imbalance, while someone else might deal with multiple. Here's a closer look at how estrogen imbalance manifests and what it might indicate:

Signs of Estrogen Dominance (Too Much Estrogen)

Estrogen dominance often occurs when your progesterone levels are too low relative to estrogen. This state can develop even if overall estrogen levels have already started to decline. Here are some signs to watch for:

- **Breast tenderness**: Hormones like estrogen can overstimulate breast tissue, causing discomfort.
- **Weight gain**: Excess estrogen is connected to fat storage, particularly around the hips, thighs, and abdomen.
- **Mood swings**: Elevated estrogen can influence serotonin and dopamine, causing irritability or unexplained highs and lows.
- **Heavy or irregular periods**: Estrogen dominance often overstimulates the uterine lining, leading to prolonged or painful periods.
- **Bloating**: High estrogen levels can cause water retention and digestive discomfort.

Tip: Track symptoms monthly to identify patterns. Symptoms that worsen in the luteal phase (the week before your period) often point to progesterone-related imbalances.

Signs of Estrogen Deficiency (Too Little Estrogen)

Estrogen deficiency usually becomes prominent during menopause due to the drop in ovarian hormone production. Symptoms include:

- *Vaginal dryness*: A common issue that can make sex uncomfortable or lead to increased risk of infections.
- *Hot flashes and night sweats*: Sudden temperature changes occur as the body adjusts to dwindling estrogen.
- *Sleep problems*: Estrogen helps regulate melatonin, so reduced levels can lead to insomnia or disrupted sleep.
- *Skin changes*: Collagen production drops, making skin thinner, less elastic, and more prone to wrinkles.
- *Bone health issues*: Low estrogen impairs bone remodeling, increasing the risk of osteoporosis and fractures.

Practical Insight: If you notice these symptoms, foods like almonds, sesame seeds, flaxseeds, and other phytoestrogen-rich options can provide gentle, natural support to mimic estrogen's action in the body.

Estrogen Dominance vs. Estrogen Deficiency

Understanding whether you're dealing with excess estrogen or insufficient estrogen helps you choose the right solutions. While it may seem counterintuitive, these conditions can overlap. For example, estrogen dominance may lead to a decline in estrogen over time due to stress on the endocrine system.

Estrogen Dominance

Estrogen dominance occurs when estrogen is high compared to progesterone. This doesn't necessarily mean your estrogen levels are high; progesterone may simply be too low.

Underlying Causes:

- Chronic stress (reduces progesterone production)
- Poor liver function (impairs estrogen detoxification)
- Exposure to xenoestrogens (chemicals that mimic estrogen in the body)
- Obesity (fat cells produce estrogen)

Strategies to Address It:

- *Focus on detoxifying foods*, like cruciferous vegetables (broccoli, cauliflower, cabbage), which support estrogen metabolism in the liver.
- *Improve gut health* by eating plenty of fiber and fermented foods. Regular bowel movements ensure

excess estrogen is flushed out instead of being reabsorbed.

Limit alcohol, as it stresses the liver and contributes to poor estrogen clearance.

Estrogen Deficiency

Women experience estrogen deficiency more commonly during and after menopause, but other factors like overexercise, being underweight, or certain medications can cause it too.

Underlying Causes:

- Menopause and age-related ovarian decline
- Low body fat percentage (since fat tissue produces estrogen post-menopause)
- High-intensity exercise without adequate recovery

Strategies to Address It:

- *Introduce phytoestrogen foods*, such as flaxseeds, lentils, and tofu. These natural compounds mimic estrogen in a much weaker form and can reduce symptoms like hot flashes.
- Consider *supplementing with omega-3 fatty acids*, which can mitigate inflammation, support brain health, and improve hormone production.

- Practice gentle exercise, such as yoga or tai chi, avoiding high-intensity activity that could further lower estrogen levels.

By identifying your specific hormonal needs and tailoring your approach accordingly, you can create a more balanced, energized, and harmonious plan for long-term wellness.

How Food Affects Hormones After 40

Hormones are highly sensitive to what you eat. After 40, your body's ability to maintain hormonal homeostasis (balance) becomes more delicate. Nutritional choices can either work to support this balance or create more disruption. This is because certain foods influence the production, regulation, and detoxification of hormones like estrogen, progesterone, and cortisol.

Key Ways Food Impacts Hormones:

1. *Nutrient Availability*: Your body needs specific nutrients to produce hormones. For example, healthy fats like omega-3s are essential for building sex hormones, while proteins are crucial for enzymes that regulate hormonal activity.
2. *Blood Sugar Stability*: Spikes and crashes in blood sugar from processed or sugary foods trigger an overproduction of insulin, a hormone that stores energy. Chronic insulin surges can lead to fat storage, disrupt estrogen balance, and increase inflammation.

Tip: Focus on complex carbohydrates like quinoa or sweet potatoes that release energy slowly.

3. *Inflammation Control*: Eating anti-inflammatory foods, like leafy greens and fatty fish, can help control cortisol (a stress hormone) and reduce strain on the hormonal system. Conversely, pro-inflammatory foods like processed meats or excessive sugar can worsen hormonal imbalances.
4. *Detoxification Support*: Your liver plays a vital role in breaking down and detoxifying hormones like estrogen after they've served their purpose. Without the right nutrients (like those found in cruciferous vegetables), this process can slow down, causing hormones to linger in the bloodstream.

Takeaway: The right foods can nurture hormonal health by stabilizing blood sugar, reducing stress, and supporting detoxification.

Estrogen-Supportive Nutrients

Specific nutrients are particularly beneficial for women over 40 as they directly support estrogen production, metabolism, and balance.

1. **Phytoestrogens:**

   Phytoestrogens are plant-derived compounds with weak estrogen-like effects. They're particularly useful during perimenopause and menopause, as they can mimic estrogen in a gentle way to reduce symptoms like hot flashes or dryness.

Examples:

- Flaxseeds (highest source of lignans, a type of phytoestrogen)
- Soy (edamame, tofu, tempeh)
- Sesame seeds
- Chickpeas and lentils

Practical Tip: Sprinkle ground flaxseeds on your oatmeal or blend it into a smoothie for a phytoestrogen boost.

2. **Omega-3 Fatty Acids:**

These healthy fats reduce inflammation and support hormone production. They can also help improve mood and combat anxiety, which often accompany hormonally driven changes.

Sources:

- Salmon, sardines, mackerel
- Chia seeds, walnuts
- Fish oil supplements

3. **Magnesium:**

Magnesium is important for managing stress and aiding good sleep, both of which are key for hormone stability. It's also involved in estrogen detoxification.

Sources:

- Spinach, Swiss chard
- Dark chocolate (opt for 70% or higher)
- Almonds

4. **B Vitamins:**

B vitamins like B6 and B12 assist in producing and metabolizing hormones. They're especially important for energy levels, brain health, and managing mood swings.

Sources:

- Eggs
- Avocados
- Fortified nutritional yeast

5. **Fiber:**

Dietary fiber helps your body remove excess estrogen by binding to it and carrying it out through digestion. Regular bowel movements are essential for eliminating "used" hormones instead of recycling them.

Sources:

- Oats
- Apples, pears
- Legumes

Foods that Help vs. Foods that Harm

Your food choices can either support hormone balance or throw it off track. Here's a breakdown of helpful options and those to avoid:

Foods that Help:

1. ***Leafy Greens and Cruciferous Vegetables***: Broccoli, kale, cabbage, and Brussels sprouts aid estrogen detoxification and provide antioxidants.
2. ***Healthy Fats***: Avocados, olive oil, and nuts provide essential building blocks for hormones.
3. ***Fermented Foods (for gut health)***: Yogurt, kimchi, sauerkraut, and kefir support a healthy microbiome, which influences estrogen metabolism.
4. ***High-Fiber Foods***: Fruits, vegetables, legumes, and whole grains support hormone regulation and digestion.

Foods that Harm:

1. ***Refined Sugars and Carbs***: They spike insulin, cause energy crashes, and inflame the body, which impacts hormonal stability. Replace these with whole food sources like fruit or sweet potatoes.

2. ***Caffeine Excess***: Too much coffee increases cortisol (stress hormone) levels, which can throw off other hormones. Switch to green tea or herbal teas like chamomile during your most stressed periods.
3. ***Alcohol***: Alcohol slows liver detoxification, which is vital for clearing unused estrogen. Limit to 1-2 servings per week or switch to non-alcoholic kombucha for digestive and hormone-friendly benefits.
4. ***Processed Foods***: Additives, preservatives, and unhealthy fats disrupt the body's natural processes. Replace packaged snacks with simple, nutrient-dense options like nuts, seeds, or vegetables with hummus.

The Role of Gut Health in Hormone Balance

Your gut might not seem like it plays a big role in hormone balance, but the truth is, it's a powerful player. A specialized group of bacteria in your gut, often called the estrobolome, helps metabolize and regulate estrogen levels in the body. When this system is imbalanced, it can lead to estrogen dominance, deficiency, or erratic hormones.

Symptoms Indicating Poor Gut Health:
- Bloating or gas
- Constipation or diarrhea
- Persistent fatigue
- Skin issues (like acne or eczema)
- Food intolerances or sensitivities

How to Support a Healthy Gut for Balanced Hormones:

1. *Prebiotic Foods*: Boost beneficial bacteria with prebiotics found in foods like garlic, onions, leeks, bananas, and asparagus. These act as "fertilizer" for good gut microbes.
2. *Probiotic Sources*: Rebuild your gut microbiome using probiotics, which introduce healthy strains of bacteria. Kefir, miso soup, and kombucha are easy additions to a meal plan.
3. *Limit Gut Disruptors*: Certain foods, such as sugar, artificial sweeteners, and alcohol, harm gut lining and suppress healthy bacteria levels. Consuming these in excess disrupts hormone processing in the gut.
4. *Hydration*: Keep digestion smooth by drinking plenty of water. A hydrated digestive tract supports the efficient elimination of waste, including excess estrogen.

Taking care of your gut is not just about digestion; it's also about creating a hormonal landscape that keeps your body functioning smoothly.

The Lifestyle Factors that Impact Estrogen

Estrogen plays a vital role in women's health, influencing energy, mood, weight, and overall well-being. However, your lifestyle choices, from how much you sleep to the products you use, can impact your estrogen levels. This guide breaks down key lifestyle factors that affect estrogen and offers actionable tips to help you maintain hormonal balance.

Sleep, Stress, and Cortisol

How Sleep and Stress Affect Estrogen

Poor sleep and chronic stress can disrupt your body's delicate hormonal balance. Sleep deprivation often leads to higher cortisol levels, which can suppress estrogen production and exacerbate symptoms like fatigue, irritability, and irregular cycles. Chronic stress triggers your body's "fight or flight" response, increasing cortisol and throwing off hormone regulation.

Tips for Restorative Sleep

- **Stick to a Schedule**: Aim to go to bed and wake up at the same time every day. A regular routine helps regulate your body's internal clock.
- **Create a Sleep Sanctuary**: Block out noise and light with blackout curtains and white noise machines. Keep your bedroom cool and clutter-free for a calming environment.
- **Nighttime Rituals**: Wind down with calming activities like reading, journaling, or practicing mindfulness. Avoid screens at least an hour before bed to reduce blue light exposure.
- **Avoid Stimulants**: Limit caffeine intake in the afternoon and avoid heavy meals or alcohol close to bedtime.

Managing Stress to Lower Cortisol

- **Breathwork Exercises**: Practice deep or diaphragmatic breathing to instantly reduce cortisol levels. Try breathing in for four counts, holding for four, and exhaling for six counts for five minutes daily.
- **Mindfulness Practices**: Incorporate yoga or meditation to build emotional resilience and combat daily stress. Even a 10-minute session can lower cortisol.
- **Set Firm Boundaries**: Whether it's saying "no" to overcommitting or planning downtime, setting boundaries can help you prioritize your well-being.

- ***Prioritize Joy***: Make time for activities you love and spend time with people who lift your energy. Modern-day busyness can often crowd out simple joys that keep you centered.

Balancing sleep and managing stress are essential for maintaining healthy cortisol levels and supporting hormonal harmony. By prioritizing restorative habits and mindfulness, you can promote overall well-being and reduce the impact of daily stressors.

Exercise that Supports Hormonal Health

Exercise plays a significant role in balancing hormones, including estrogen. Moderate activity helps regulate body weight, which affects estrogen since fat tissues can produce estrogen on their own. However, intense exercise or overtraining can strain your body and lead to disruptions in hormone production.

Types of Exercise to Incorporate

1. **Strength Training:**
   Building muscle not only enhances your physical strength but also boosts insulin sensitivity, which can help regulate blood sugar levels and promote hormonal balance. Exercises like weightlifting, using resistance bands, or bodyweight workouts such as push-ups and squats are great options. Aim to include strength

training sessions twice a week, focusing on different muscle groups each time for well-rounded benefits.

2. **Low-Impact Cardio**

Cardiovascular activities like walking, cycling, swimming, or gentle aerobics improve heart health, boost circulation, and increase endurance without placing excessive strain on your joints. These exercises are especially beneficial if you're looking for a sustainable and less intense way to stay active. For best results, aim for at least 150 minutes of moderate cardio per week, or break it into manageable sessions throughout your week.

3. **Restorative Movement**

High-energy workouts are great, but balancing them with restorative practices like yoga, pilates, or tai chi is essential for maintaining overall well-being. These low-intensity activities calm the nervous system, reduce stress, improve posture, and enhance flexibility. They also promote better breathing and mindfulness, allowing you to recharge mentally while staying active physically.

4. **Find Your Rhythm**

Exercise doesn't have to leave you feeling drained. If you often feel depleted after workouts, consider lowering the intensity or shortening the duration. Tune into your body's signals and adjust as needed.

Adding regular rest or recovery days to your routine can help prevent overtraining, reduce the risk of injury, and keep your energy levels consistent, ensuring long-term success in staying active.

Balancing exercise with your body's needs is key to supporting hormonal health and overall well-being. By combining strength training, low-impact cardio, and restorative movement, you can create a sustainable routine that promotes balance and vitality.

Environmental Toxins and Estrogen Disruptors

Certain chemicals mimic the effects of estrogen, leading to imbalances like estrogen dominance. These synthetic estrogens, called xenoestrogens, are found in everyday items like plastics, cleaning supplies, and personal care products. Over time, exposure to these toxins burdens your liver and creates hormonal disruption.

How to Minimize Toxin Exposure

1. **Rethink Plastics**

   Single-use plastics are not just harmful to the environment—they can also impact your health. Avoid using them whenever possible and opt for reusable alternatives like glass, stainless steel, or silicone containers for food and drink storage.

For added safety, avoid microwaving food in plastic containers, as heat can cause harmful chemicals like BPA and phthalates to leach into your food. Small changes, like switching to reusable shopping bags or beeswax wraps, can also make a big difference.

2. **Upgrade Your Personal Care Routine**

Many personal care products contain hidden chemicals that can disrupt your hormones or irritate your skin. When shopping, read labels carefully and steer clear of ingredients like parabens, phthalates, and synthetic fragrances.

These can be found in everything from shampoos to lotions. Instead, look for clean beauty brands marked "paraben-free," "phthalate-free," or "fragrance-free," which offer safer alternatives. Switching to natural deodorants, sulfate-free shampoos, and organic skincare products is a great start.

3. **Switch to Natural Cleaning Products**

Conventional cleaning products often contain harsh chemicals that can harm your health and pollute the environment. Swap them out for eco-friendly alternatives like vinegar-based cleaners, baking soda for scrubbing, or products certified as non-toxic and biodegradable.

Not only are these options safer for your family, but they're also gentler on the planet. Plus, many DIY recipes use simple ingredients like lemon and essential oils to leave your home fresh and clean.

4. Use Filtered Water

Tap water may appear clean, but it can contain contaminants such as pesticides, heavy metals, microplastics, and even hormone residues. Installing a high-quality water filter for your drinking water and cooking needs can help reduce these impurities. Options like carbon filters, reverse osmosis systems, or faucet-mounted filters can provide safer and better-tasting water for the whole family.

5. Non-Toxic Cookware

The cookware you choose can directly affect your health. Non-stick coatings like Teflon can release toxic fumes when overheated, which can be harmful over time. Instead, opt for safer options like ceramic, cast iron, or stainless steel.

These materials are durable, easy to clean, and free from harmful chemicals. For baking, use uncoated stainless steel or glass pans to avoid exposure to toxins. Investing in healthy cookware not only protects your meals but also ensures long-lasting kitchen tools.

You don't need to overhaul everything at once! Start where it feels easiest, like swapping plastic water bottles for glass or editing your personal care routine. These small, consistent changes will reduce your toxin exposure over time.

Your lifestyle has a profound impact on your hormonal health, with factors like sleep, stress, exercise, and toxin exposure playing critical roles. By improving your sleep hygiene, managing stress, staying active, and reducing environmental toxins, you can support healthy estrogen levels and overall hormone balance.

Remember, you don't need to be perfect to see improvements. Start with small, manageable changes and build from there. Whether it's taking five minutes to breathe deeply, switching to safer cleaning products, or introducing regular strength training, every positive action contributes to a healthier, more balanced you.

Planning Your Hormone-Smart Kitchen

The kitchen is the heart of your home and the foundation of a hormone-supportive lifestyle. By stocking it with the right pantry essentials, planning your meals strategically, and being mindful of hidden hormone disruptors, you can set yourself up for success.

A hormone-smart kitchen empowers you to make nutritious choices easily, create balanced meals, and reduce exposure to toxins that could interfere with your health. Here's how to plan, stock, and prep with your hormones in mind.

Pantry Essentials and Grocery List

A hormone-smart kitchen starts with the right ingredients. Focus on stocking whole, nutrient-dense foods that naturally support estrogen balance, nourish your gut microbiome, and reduce inflammation. Simplify your grocery shopping with a carefully curated list that includes the essentials for hormonal health.

Hormone-Smart Pantry Staples

1. **Whole Grains and Fiber-Rich Foods:**

   Fiber helps eliminate excess estrogen and supports gut health.

   - Quinoa
   - Brown rice
   - Oats
   - Barley
   - Whole-grain pasta

2. **Healthy Fats:**

   These are the building blocks of hormone production.

   - Extra virgin olive oil
   - Coconut oil (for cooking at higher temperatures)
   - Avocados
   - Nut butters (like almond or cashew butter)
   - Chia seeds, flaxseeds, and hemp seeds

3. **Plant-Based Proteins and Legumes:**

   Rich in phytoestrogens, fiber, and essential amino acids.

   - Lentils
   - Chickpeas
   - Black beans
   - Edamame

4. **Nuts and Seeds:**

Packed with magnesium, fatty acids, and hormonal support properties.

- Walnuts
- Almonds
- Sunflower seeds
- Pumpkin seeds

5. **Spices and Herbs:**

Spices aren't just flavorful; they provide anti-inflammatory and detoxifying benefits.

- Turmeric (curcumin aids liver detoxification)
- Cinnamon (helps balance blood sugar levels)
- Ginger (anti-inflammatory properties)
- Garlic (prebiotic benefits for gut health)

Refrigerator and Freezer Essentials

1. **Fresh Produce:**

Focus on a colorful variety to ensure you're getting a wide range of nutrients.

- Cruciferous vegetables (broccoli, kale, cauliflower, cabbage)
- Leafy greens (spinach, Swiss chard, arugula)
- Berries (blueberries, raspberries, strawberries)
- Citrus fruits (oranges, lemons, grapefruits)
- Sweet potatoes and carrots

2. **Proteins:**
    - Organic, free-range eggs
    - Organic chicken or turkey
    - Fatty fish (salmon, mackerel, sardines for omega-3s)
    - Tofu and tempeh (fermented soy for phytoestrogens)
3. **Fermented Foods:**

    Support gut bacteria that help regulate estrogen.

    - Yogurt (opt for unsweetened, live-culture brands)
    - Kimchi or sauerkraut
    - Miso paste
4. **Freezer Staples:**

    Stock up on frozen fruits and vegetables for convenience. Look for options without sauces or additives.

    - Frozen spinach, peas, and broccoli
    - Frozen berries for smoothies
    - Pre-cooked quinoa or rice

Example Grocery List

Use this list as a foundation and adjust it to your eating preferences:

1. Fresh kale and spinach

2. Organic eggs
3. A bag of quinoa
4. Cans of chickpeas and black beans
5. Olive oil and almond butter
6. Fresh salmon or mackerel
7. Flaxseeds and chia seeds
8. Unsweetened Greek yogurt
9. Frozen mixed berries
10. Fresh ginger and garlic

Stocking your kitchen with hormone-smart essentials is a simple yet powerful way to support your overall health. With these nutrient-packed staples, you can create balanced, nourishing meals that promote hormone balance and well-being.

How to Meal Prep with Hormones in Mind

Meal prepping is one of the most effective ways to stay on track with your hormonal health goals. By dedicating a couple of hours each week to prepping meals and snacks, you save time, avoid decision fatigue, and set yourself up with balanced options that support your well-being.

1. **Plan Your Meals for the Week**

    Before you start cooking, create a simple plan for your week.

- ***Structure Meals Around Hormonal Balance***: Pair healthy fats, lean protein, and fiber-rich carbs at every meal to keep blood sugar levels stable and support hormone production.
- ***Include Cruciferous Vegetables Daily***: Aim for at least one serving of broccoli, kale, or cabbage each day to aid in estrogen detoxification.
- ***Rotate Your Proteins***: Alternate between plant-based options (like tofu or lentils) and lean animal proteins (like chicken or fish) to ensure variety.

Example Weekly Meal Plan

- ***Breakfasts***: Smoothies with berries, spinach, flaxseeds, and almond milk; or avocado toast with boiled eggs.
- ***Lunches***: Grain bowls with quinoa, roasted vegetables, and tahini dressing; or green salads with grilled chicken and a handful of nuts.
- ***Dinners***: Baked salmon with roasted Brussels sprouts and brown rice; or a stir-fry with tofu, broccoli, and sesame oil.

2. **Batch Cook for Convenience**

Batch cooking allows you to have staples ready to mix and match throughout the week.

- ***Cook a Large Batch of Grains***: Prep quinoa, brown rice, or farro to use as the base for salads or bowls.
- ***Roast a Tray of Vegetables***: Use olive oil, salt, and spices to roast broccoli, zucchini, and sweet potatoes for easy sides.
- ***Prepare a Protein of Choice***: Grill chicken breasts, bake a piece of salmon, or cook a pot of lentils.

3. **Pre-Portion Snacks**

Hormone-friendly snacks help you avoid blood sugar spikes between meals.

- Pack small containers of nuts or trail mix.
- Pre-cut fresh veggies like carrot sticks or celery and pair with hummus.
- Portion out servings of yogurt with berries or granola on the side.

4. **Use Freezer-Friendly Options**

Make double portions of meals and freeze extras for busier days. Soups, stews, and casseroles freeze well and are easy to reheat.

Meal prepping with hormones in mind can make a huge difference in maintaining balance and supporting overall health. With a little planning and preparation, you can save time, reduce stress, and nourish your body with meals that work for you all week long.

Reading Labels and Avoiding Hidden Estrogen Disruptors

While choosing hormone-friendly foods is essential, it's equally important to be mindful of the hidden chemicals and additives that can sneak into your meals. Many processed foods and everyday products contain xenoestrogens, synthetic compounds that mimic estrogen and disrupt hormonal balance.

Understanding Common Label Pitfalls

1. *Added Sugar*: Excessive sugar consumption raises insulin levels, which can indirectly impact estrogen. Be wary of foods labeled as "low fat," as these often compensate for flavor by adding sugar.
    - Look Out For: Ingredients like high-fructose corn syrup, maltose, and dextrose.
2. *Preservatives and Artificial Additives*: Chemical preservatives like BPA, found in canned foods and plastic packaging, can leach into food and act as endocrine disruptors.
    - Opt For: BPA-free cans or fresh and frozen alternatives.

3. ***Synthetic Hormones in Animal Products***: Non-organic dairy and meat products may contain added hormones or antibiotics.
    - Choose: Organic, grass-fed, or hormone-free options whenever possible.
4. ***Hidden Oils and Fats***: Refined oils like soybean or canola oil are often found in processed foods and contribute to inflammation.
    - Stick To: Whole-food fats such as olive oil or avocado oil.

How to Read Labels Like a Pro

- ***Check Ingredient Length***: If the list includes ingredients you can't pronounce or recognize, it's a red flag.
- ***Prioritize Whole Foods***: Products should contain minimal, real ingredients (e.g., "almonds" instead of "almond flavor").
- ***Watch for Buzzwords***: "Natural" and "healthy" don't necessarily mean hormone-friendly. Always read the full label.

By thoughtfully planning, stocking, and prepping in your kitchen, you create a supportive environment for hormonal balance. Investing a little time and attention into these habits will not only improve your immediate health but set a strong foundation for long-term wellness.

Your 3-Week Estrogen Diet Plan

Supporting hormonal balance through diet isn't just about restrictive eating—it's about providing your body with the nourishment it needs to function optimally. This 3-week plan is designed to gently guide you through the key phases of hormonal health transformation.

Each week builds on the last, offering targeted strategies that nourish your body, calm your mind, and restore balance. By the end of the three weeks, you'll have established a sustainable, hormone-friendly routine that supports your well-being now and in the future.

Week 1: Clean Out, Calm Down, Reset

This week is all about giving your body a fresh start. Think of it as a detox for both your body and mind. By cutting out common hormone disruptors and adding food and habits that support your hormones, you'll begin to feel more balanced and clear-headed by the end of the week. Take it one day at a time, and don't worry about being perfect. Small, intentional steps are what matter most.

Goals for Week 1

- Eliminate foods and habits that may disrupt your hormones.
- Calm inflammation and support your body's natural detox processes.
- Start a solid foundation for renewed energy, better sleep, and fewer hormone-related symptoms.

Foods to Avoid During Week 1

- Processed foods (chips, fast food, pre-packaged meals).
- Sugars (cut out candy, sodas, sweetened yogurt, and pastries).
- Alcohol (which disrupts sleep and puts stress on your liver).
- Refined carbohydrates (like white bread, white rice, and sugary cereals).

Focus on fresh, whole foods that nourish your body, and drink plenty of water to stay hydrated each day.

Day 1

Morning:

- Drink a cup of warm lemon water to wake up your digestion.
- Enjoy a green smoothie packed with hormone-friendly ingredients:

- Handful of spinach
- 1 tablespoon ground flaxseeds
- ½ cup frozen berries (blueberries or raspberries)
- 1 cup unsweetened almond milk
- Optional: A scoop of protein powder (check for clean, sugar-free options).

Mid-Morning Snack:

- A small handful of unsalted nuts like almonds or walnuts. These contain healthy fats to stabilize your blood sugar.

Lunch:

- A warm bowl of lentil and vegetable soup. Lentils are rich in fiber and phytoestrogens, which aid in balancing estrogen. Pair the soup with a simple side salad of arugula dressed with olive oil and lemon.

Afternoon Tip:

- Take 10 minutes to stretch or sit quietly and focus on deep breathing. This helps lower cortisol (a stress hormone that can disrupt others).

Dinner:

- Grilled wild-caught salmon with steamed broccoli and roasted sweet potato cubes drizzled in olive oil.

Broccoli supports your liver, helping it detoxify old estrogen.

Evening Wind-Down:

- Sip on chamomile tea before bed to promote calmness. Try journaling or reading to relax and prepare for sleep.

Day 2

Morning:

- Overnight oats topped with chia seeds, cinnamon, and fresh apple slices. Chia seeds are full of omega-3s, which combat inflammation and support brain function.

Mid-Morning Snack:

- Sliced cucumber with 2 tablespoons of hummus. This light snack gives you hydration and plant-based nutrients.

Lunch:

- A large mixed greens salad with grilled chicken, sliced avocado, sunflower seeds, and a drizzle of olive oil and balsamic vinegar. Add a sprinkle of flaxseeds for extra fiber.

Activity Tip:

- Take a 20-minute walk outside. Exposure to natural light helps regulate your circadian rhythm (critical for hormone health).

Dinner:

- Stir-fried tofu with broccoli, red bell peppers, and snap peas over a bed of quinoa. Flavor it with a splash of tamari or coconut aminos, which are low-sodium alternatives to soy sauce.

Evening Wind-Down:

- Dedicate just 5-10 minutes before bed for deep breathing or mindfulness meditation. It'll help lower cortisol levels and relax your nervous system.

Day 3

Morning:

- Start your day with a cup of warm lemon water, followed by scrambled eggs cooked with spinach and a side of two slices of avocado.

Mid-Morning Snack:

- A green apple with almond butter (1 tablespoon). This snack keeps your energy steady without spiking your blood sugar.

Lunch:

- A warming bowl of quinoa salad tossed with black beans, shredded carrots, chopped parsley, and a simple lime-tahini dressing.

Hydration Reminder:

- Enhance your water by adding fresh mint leaves or cucumber slices for flavor. Aim for at least 6-8 glasses of water today.

Dinner:

- Baked cod or halibut served with a mix of roasted Brussels sprouts and butternut squash. The fiber and antioxidants in these veggies help reduce inflammation.

Evening Tip:

- Swap your evening screen time with a calming activity, like reading, light yoga, or listening to soothing music.

Day 4 through Day 7

The second half of the week focuses on consistency. Rotate your meals to keep things interesting, but stick to clean, whole foods and avoid the "toxic four" (sugar, alcohol, processed food, and refined carbs).

Morning Options:

- Green smoothie with flaxseeds and frozen berries.
- Chia seed pudding with unsweetened coconut milk and fresh fruit.
- Scrambled eggs with sautéed leafy greens like kale or spinach.

Mid-Morning Snacks:

- Raw veggies with guacamole.
- Pumpkin seeds or roasted chickpeas.
- A hard-boiled egg paired with an orange or a handful of blueberries.

Lunch Options:

- Lentil soup with a side of steamed asparagus.
- Mixed greens salad with grilled salmon, walnuts, and a mustard vinaigrette.
- Turkey lettuce wraps with shredded carrots, cucumber, and tahini dressing.

Afternoon Boost:

- Listen to your body's cues for stress or fatigue. If you're feeling overwhelmed, take 5 minutes to sit quietly and deep breathe, focusing on longer exhales.

Dinner Options:

- Stir-fried tofu or shrimp with zucchini noodles and a sesame glaze.

- Grilled chicken breast served with roasted carrots and sautéed spinach.
- Wild-caught fish over a bed of wild or brown rice with a lemon-herb dressing.

Evening Self-Care Tips:

- Add Epsom salt to a warm bath to relax your muscles and increase magnesium.
- Reflect on your wins for the day, such as choosing water over soda or stepping outdoors for fresh air.

Weekly Lifestyle Tips:

- Don't obsess over calories; focus on nourishing your body with whole, unprocessed foods.
- Prioritize sleep as a reset for your hormones. Create a nighttime routine to wind down, like dimming lights and avoiding screens an hour before bedtime.
- Practice saying "no" to demands that overwhelm you, even if that means skipping unnecessary tasks.

At the end of Week 1, you'll feel lighter, more energized, and ready to tackle Week 2, which will focus on bringing in even more nourishing foods to balance and stabilize your hormones. Keep taking it one day at a time, and trust that these small shifts are making a big difference!

Week 2: Nourish and Balance

This week, we're building on the clean foundation from Week 1 by focusing on adding nutrient-rich, hormone-loving foods into your meals. The key word here is balance. You'll prioritize eating whole, unprocessed meals that support steady blood sugar, promote estrogen metabolism, and keep you feeling energized throughout the day.

Goals for Week 2

1. Add foods rich in phytoestrogens, fiber, and healthy fats.
2. Stabilize energy levels by eating regularly and balancing macronutrients at every meal.
3. Develop easy-to-follow meal planning habits for long-term success.

Day 8

Morning:

- Start your day with scrambled eggs cooked in olive oil, mixed with sautéed spinach. Add two slices of avocado on the side for healthy fats.
- **Tip**: Eggs are not only protein-packed but also contain choline, a nutrient that supports brain health, which is important during hormonal changes.

Mid-Morning Snack:

- A crunchy green apple with 1 tablespoon of almond butter.

Lunch:

- A quinoa and black bean salad. Combine cooked quinoa, black beans, cherry tomatoes, fresh cilantro, and a simple lime-tahini dressing. Add a handful of mixed greens as a base for an extra nutrient boost.

Hydration Tip:

- Jazz up your water by adding cucumber slices, fresh mint, or a squeeze of lemon. Aim for at least 8 glasses per day to support hydration and digestion.

Dinner:

- Grilled chicken thighs with oven-roasted Brussels sprouts (lightly tossed in olive oil and garlic) and steamed carrots on the side.

Wind-Down:

- Take 10-15 minutes before bed to stretch or do a light yoga session. This relaxes your muscles and preps your mind for restful sleep.

Day 9

Morning:

- Blend a green smoothie with kale, unsweetened coconut milk, 1 tablespoon flaxseeds, ½ a banana, and ½ cup frozen pineapple. This phytoestrogen-rich breakfast is packed with fiber and antioxidants.

Mid-Morning Snack:

- 1 boiled egg and ½ an avocado lightly sprinkled with sea salt.

Lunch:

- Turkey lettuce wraps. Fill large romaine leaves with sliced turkey, shredded carrots, thinly sliced cucumber, and tahini spread. Pair with a handful of raw veggies like celery and bell peppers as a crunchy side.

Activity Tip:

- Take 10-15 minutes to add a strength-building session. Simple exercises like squats, resistance band work, or light dumbbells help regulate insulin and balance hormones.

Dinner:

- Lentil and veggie curry served over brown rice. Include turmeric and ginger during cooking to boost anti-inflammatory benefits.

Stress-Busting Ritual:

- Dedicate a few minutes before bed to journaling. Write down three things you're grateful for to shift your mindset to positivity and help manage stress.

Day 10

Morning:

- Overnight chia seed pudding made with unsweetened almond milk, topped with fresh strawberries and a handful of pistachios.

Mid-Morning Snack:

- A boiled egg and added crunch from raw carrot sticks.

Lunch:

- Tossed greens with roasted chickpeas, sliced avocado, cherry tomatoes, sunflower seeds, and a lemon-olive oil vinaigrette.

Afternoon Reminder:

- Practice mindfulness for 5 minutes while sitting comfortably. Focus on your breath to reset your nervous system and lower cortisol.

Dinner:

- Baked cod served with roasted zucchini and sweet potato wedges. Squeeze a bit of fresh lemon over the fish before serving for brightness.

Evening Wind-Down:

- Spend 15 minutes reading a book or doing deep breathing exercises instead of using screens before bed.

Day 11 through Day 14

For the remaining days of the week, maintain steady blood sugar by eating balanced meals every 3-4 hours. Rotate from different meal ideas and continue focusing on nutrient-dense foods.

Morning Options:

- An omelet stuffed with spinach, mushrooms, and a sprinkle of goat cheese.
- A smoothie made with frozen peaches, flaxseeds, and coconut water.
- Chia pudding with coconut milk, cinnamon, and fresh berries.

Mid-Morning Snacks for Variety:

- A small handful of raw nuts (like cashews or almonds).
- Raw cucumber slices or sugar snap peas with hummus.
- Greek yogurt (unsweetened) topped with a sprinkle of ground flaxseeds.

Lunch Options:

- Roasted beet and arugula salad with grilled salmon.
- A quinoa veggie bowl topped with tahini dressing and a handful of spinach.
- Miso soup with a side of steamed edamame and sliced avocado.

Dinner Ideas:

- Stir-fried shrimp with bok choy, asparagus, and red peppers in a sesame ginger glaze over brown rice.
- Grilled turkey burger patties served with a side of avocado and roasted cauliflower.
- Stuffed bell peppers filled with a mix of quinoa, lentils, diced tomatoes, and onions.

Activity Suggestions for Days 11-14:

- Include light resistance training 2-3 times this week to improve muscle tone and metabolic health.
- Dedicate 10-15 minutes daily to mindfulness or meditation. Try guided meditation apps if you're new to the practice.

Evening Routines:

- Set a calming environment before bed. Dimming lights 1-2 hours before sleep signals to your body that it's time to wind down.

- Pair an herbal tea like spearmint or chamomile with a cozy evening ritual, such as journaling or light stretching.

Lifestyle Reminders for Week 2

- Continue avoiding sugar, alcohol, and refined carbs to stabilize your energy levels and prevent hormonal spikes.
- Support your liver by including at least one cruciferous vegetable daily (e.g., broccoli, kale, cabbage). These help your body detox excess estrogen naturally.
- Take note of your digestion this week. Foods like miso (fermented soy), kimchi, and plain kefir are great for improving gut health, which directly impacts hormonal balance.

By the end of Week 2, you'll not only feel more nourished and balanced but will have started building habits that make healthy hormone-supportive eating feel second nature. Week 3 will focus on fine-tuning and sustaining these healthy patterns!

Week 3: Thrive and Sustain

By now, you've begun building strong habits that support your hormones, energy, and overall well-being. Week 3 is all about refining and maintaining those shifts while introducing small tweaks that keep things fresh and exciting. The focus is to thrive through better energy levels, a calmer mind, and long-term health routines you can sustain without feeling overwhelmed.

Goals for Week 3

1. Maintain steady blood sugar and productive estrogen metabolism.
2. Build a routine you enjoy and can stick with, long-term.
3. Feel stronger, more energized, and confident in your choices.

Day 15

Morning:

- Begin your day with chia seed pudding made with unsweetened almond milk, topped with fresh strawberries and a sprinkle of pistachios. This protein-rich meal also delivers fiber and omega-3s, both important for hormonal health.

Mid-Morning Snack:

- A handful of edamame pods lightly sprinkled with sea salt. Edamame contains phytoestrogens, which can help balance estrogen levels.

Lunch:

- Grilled salmon served over a bed of arugula and shaved fennel, drizzled with a citrus vinaigrette (made of olive oil, orange juice, and a dash of mustard). This meal supports estrogen metabolism and delivers heart-healthy omega-3s.

Hydration Tip:

- Sip on peppermint tea with your lunch. It's gentle on your digestion and soothing for your stomach.

Dinner:

- Zucchini noodles topped with baked turkey meatballs and a marinara sauce made from organic tomatoes. Garnish with a sprinkle of fresh basil for extra flavor.

Evening Wind-Down:

- Spend 10 minutes journaling about your progress so far. Reflect on how you feel compared to Day 1 and note any changes in your mood, energy, or digestion.

Day 16

Morning:

- Blend a creamy smoothie with spinach, unsweetened almond milk, 1 tablespoon ground flaxseeds, half a banana, and a scoop of high-quality collagen powder. This smoothie supports skin health, joint comfort, and gut repair.

Mid-Morning Snack:

- A handful of mixed nuts and a few dark chocolate chips (85% cacao or higher). This combines healthy fats to sustain your energy and a small treat to keep things fun.

Lunch:

- A whole-grain wrap filled with hummus, roasted bell peppers, eggplant, and fresh spinach. Pair it with a small side of cucumber slices for added crunch.

Stress-Buster Tip:

- Dedicate 10 minutes after lunch to deep breathing or journaling. Simple techniques such as focusing on your breaths or jotting down what's on your mind can help reduce mid-day stress and lower cortisol.

Dinner:

- A vibrant wild rice bowl topped with shrimp, snap peas, and a sesame-ginger glaze. Wild rice adds fiber, shrimp packs in lean protein, and sesame boosts your healthy fat intake.

Evening Ritual:

- Swap evening snacks for a calming herbal tea like chamomile or spearmint. These herbs naturally promote relaxation and balance hormones.

Days 17–21

- For the rest of the week, it's time to solidify the routines that have energized and balanced your hormones so far. This is also a great opportunity to celebrate your progress and explore new variations of your favorite recipes from earlier weeks.

Morning Meal Ideas:

- Scrambled eggs with sautéed kale and a side of sweet potato cubes.
- Green smoothies with frozen mango, spinach, flaxseeds, and coconut water (refreshing and hydrating).
- Flaxseed banana bread (a fun hormone-friendly recipe).

Snack Ideas:

- Roasted chickpeas (seasoned lightly with olive oil and smoked paprika).
- Greek yogurt (unsweetened) with a small handful of flaxseeds and fresh raspberries.
- Homemade energy bites (rolled oats, almond butter, and a touch of honey).

Easy Lunches to Rotate:

- Grilled chicken salad tossed with mixed greens, avocado, roasted sweet potato chunks, and tahini-lime dressing.
- A quinoa bowl with roasted broccoli, chickpeas, and a drizzle of olive oil.
- Leftover lentil or vegetable soups from Weeks 1 and 2.

Dinner Options:

- Baked salmon served with asparagus and wild rice pilaf.
- Stir-fried tofu with red cabbage, garlic, sesame seeds, and zucchini noodles.
- A black bean taco night with hormone-friendly add-ins like guacamole and shredded lettuce (use a whole-grain or lettuce wrap).

Experiment with Recipes:

- This week, try making baked flaxseed banana bread or chickpea-stuffed sweet potatoes. These fun dishes are nutrient-dense and keep things exciting for your taste buds.

Activity Tip:

- Add more movement this week, whether it's through Pilates, swimming, or brisk walks. These low-impact exercises improve circulation, strengthen muscles, and keep your hormones balanced. Aim for about 30 minutes a day.

Evening and Sleep Routine:

- Keep consistent with your calming bedtime ritual. A warm bath with Epsom salts or lavender oil could work wonders. Make sure to dim lights an hour before bed to signal to your body that it's time to relax.

Lifestyle Reminders for Week 3

1. Focus on how foods make your body feel. If something leaves you feeling sluggish or bloated, take note, as this could be a sign your body isn't digesting it well. A food diary can help you refine your routine.
2. Keep choosing whole, minimally processed foods. Over time, you'll naturally reduce your reliance on packaged or quick-fix meals.
3. Assess your beauty and cleaning products; many contain hormone-disrupting chemicals. Aim to switch to clean options when possible.

By the end of this week, you'll have a routine that includes consistent meal prep, regular movement, and better stress management. These strategies are building blocks for long-term hormonal health, helping you thrive with more vitality and control over your well-being.

Simple Recipes for Hormone Harmony

Here are easy, nutrient-packed recipes to promote hormonal health. They are divided into breakfasts, lunches, dinners, and snacks/herbal support. Each recipe emphasizes fiber, healthy fats, lean proteins, and phytoestrogens to keep your hormones in balance.

Breakfasts

Berry & Chia Hormone-Balancing Smoothie

Ingredients:

- 1 cup unsweetened almond milk
- ½ cup frozen mixed berries
- 1 tablespoon chia seeds
- 1 scoop plant-based protein powder (optional)
- ½ tsp cinnamon

Instructions:

1. In a blender, combine all ingredients and blend until smooth.
2. Pour into a glass and enjoy!

Spinach & Mushroom Omelet

Ingredients:

- 2 organic eggs
- 1 cup baby spinach
- ¼ cup chopped mushrooms
- 1 tablespoon olive oil

Instructions:

1. In a small pan, heat olive oil over medium heat.
2. Add spinach and mushrooms to the pan and sauté until wilted.
3. In a separate bowl, whisk together eggs.
4. Pour the egg mixture into the pan with the spinach and mushrooms.
5. Cook for 2-3 minutes on one side, then flip and cook for an additional 1-2 minutes on the other side.
6. Serve hot and enjoy!

Flaxseed & Nut Butter Bowl

Ingredients:

- 1 packet steel-cut oatmeal (or ½ cup cooked)
- 1 tablespoon ground flaxseed
- 1 tablespoon almond or peanut butter
- 1 sliced banana

Instructions:

1. Cook the steel-cut oatmeal according to package instructions.
2. Once cooked, add ground flaxseed and nut butter to the hot oatmeal and stir until well combined.
3. Top with sliced banana.
4. Enjoy a healthy breakfast bowl packed with fiber, protein, and healthy fats!

Avocado Toast With Sesame Seeds

Ingredients:

- 1 slice sprouted grain bread
- ½ avocado, mashed
- 1 tsp sesame seeds
- A pinch of chili flakes and sea salt

Instructions:

1. Toast the sprouted grain bread until crispy.
2. Spread mashed avocado on top of the toast.
3. Sprinkle with sesame seeds, chili flakes, and sea salt.
4. Serve as a quick and healthy breakfast or snack option!

Phytoestrogen Smoothie Bowl

Ingredients:

- ½ cup plain coconut yogurt
- 1 tablespoon ground flaxseeds
- ½ cup frozen strawberries
- ⅓ cup cooked quinoa (cooled)
- 1 tsp honey (optional)

Instructions:

1. In a blender, combine the coconut yogurt, ground flaxseeds, frozen strawberries, cooked quinoa, and honey (if desired).
2. Blend until smooth and creamy.
3. Pour into a bowl and top with your favorite toppings such as fresh berries, sliced almonds, or shredded coconut.
4. Enjoy this delicious and nutritious smoothie bowl for breakfast or as a post-workout snack!

Lunches

Quinoa & Roasted Veggie Bowl

Ingredients:

- 1 cup cooked quinoa
- ½ cup roasted zucchini and bell peppers
- 1 tablespoon tahini dressing

Instructions:

1. Cook quinoa according to package instructions.
2. Preheat oven to 400°F and line a baking sheet with parchment paper.
3. Cut zucchini and bell peppers into bite-sized pieces and place on the prepared baking sheet.
4. Drizzle with olive oil, sprinkle with salt and pepper, and toss until evenly coated.
5. Roast in the oven for 20-25 minutes until the vegetables are tender and slightly golden.
6. Mix the cooked quinoa and roasted vegetables in a bowl, then drizzle with tahini dressing.
7. Enjoy this delicious protein-packed lunch option that is also full of fiber and healthy fats!

Hormone-Friendly Lentil Salad

Ingredients:

- 1 cup cooked lentils
- 1 cup arugula
- ½ roasted beet, diced
- Lemon juice and olive oil dressing

Instructions:

1. In a bowl, combine cooked lentils, arugula, and roasted beet.
2. Drizzle with lemon juice and olive oil dressing.
3. Toss to coat evenly.

This hormone-friendly lentil salad is packed with plant-based protein and leafy greens, making it a nutritious addition to any meal!

Tofu Collard Wrap

Ingredients:

- 2 large collard green leaves
- ¼ cup baked tofu strips
- ¼ cup shredded carrots
- 1 tablespoon hummus

Instructions:

1. Lay collard green leaves flat on a cutting board.
2. Spread hummus evenly on each leaf.
3. Place tofu strips and shredded carrots in the middle of the leaves.
4. Roll up tightly, tucking in the sides as you go.
5. Slice into bite-sized pieces or enjoy whole for a filling and nutritious lunch.

Collard greens are rich in antioxidants and provide a great alternative to traditional wraps made with refined flour tortillas.

Mediterranean Chickpea Bowl

Ingredients:

- ½ cup cooked chickpeas
- 1 cup mixed greens
- 4 cherry tomatoes, halved
- 1 tablespoon olive oil
- A sprinkle of sesame seeds

Instructions:

1. Start by prepping your chickpeas. You can use canned chickpeas or cook them yourself. If using canned, drain and rinse well.
2. In a bowl, combine the cooked chickpeas with olive oil and sesame seeds.
3. Heat a pan over medium heat and add in the chickpea mixture. Cook for about 5 minutes, until slightly crispy.
4. Meanwhile, assemble your bowl by adding mixed greens and cherry tomatoes on a bed of rice or quinoa.
5. Once the chickpeas are ready, add them to the bowl on top of the greens and tomatoes.
6. Optional toppings: sliced avocado, feta cheese, hummus drizzle.

Sweet Potato & Spinach Wrap

Ingredients:

- 1 whole-grain wrap
- ½ cup roasted sweet potatoes, cubed
- 1 cup sautéed spinach
- 1 tablespoon tahini

Instructions:

1. Preheat a pan over medium heat.
2. Warm up the whole-grain wrap for about 30 seconds on each side.
3. Spread tahini evenly on the wrap.
4. Add sautéed spinach and roasted sweet potatoes on one half of the wrap.
5. Fold the other half over to create a wrap.
6. Place the wrap back in the pan and cook for about 2-3 minutes on each side until lightly crispy.
7. Serve with a side of fruit or salad for a complete meal.

Dinners

Grilled Salmon With Lemon & Greens

Ingredients:

- 1 salmon fillet (4 oz)
- 1 cup steamed broccoli
- 1 teaspoon olive oil
- Juice of ½ lemon

Instructions:

1. Preheat grill to medium heat.
2. Brush olive oil on both sides of the salmon fillet and sprinkle with salt and pepper.
3. Place the salmon on the grill, skin side down, and cook for about 6-8 minutes or until it flakes easily with a fork.
4. While the salmon is cooking, steam broccoli in a pot or microwave until tender.
5. Once the salmon is done, remove from grill and place onto a plate.
6. Squeeze lemon juice over the top of the salmon.
7. Serve with steamed broccoli on the side for a healthy and satisfying dinner.

Tofu Stir-Fry With Brown Rice

Ingredients:

- ½ cup cubed tofu
- 1 cup mixed stir-fry vegetables (bell peppers, snap peas, broccoli)
- 1 tablespoon coconut aminos or tamari
- ½ cup cooked brown rice

Instructions:

1. Heat a non-stick pan over medium-high heat.
2. Add cubed tofu to the pan and cook until lightly browned, about 5-7 minutes.
3. Add mixed stir-fry vegetables to the pan and cook for another 3-4 minutes until tender.
4. Pour coconut aminos or tamari over the tofu and vegetables, stirring to evenly coat everything.
5. Serve the stir-fry over cooked brown rice for a delicious and protein-packed meal.

Roasted Chicken With Root Vegetables

Ingredients:

- 1 chicken breast
- 1 cup roasted carrots and parsnips
- 1 tablespoon olive oil
- Fresh thyme or rosemary

Instructions:

1. Preheat your oven to 375°F.
2. In a baking dish, add chicken breast and drizzle with olive oil.
3. Season with fresh thyme or rosemary, salt, and pepper to taste.
4. Add in roasted carrots and parsnips around the chicken breast.
5. Bake for 25-30 minutes until the chicken is cooked through and vegetables are tender.
6. Serve hot as a hearty and comforting meal.

Lentil & Spinach One-Pot Dish

Ingredients:

- 1 cup cooked lentils
- 1 cup fresh spinach
- 1 clove minced garlic
- 1 tablespoon olive oil

Instructions:

1. In a large pot, heat olive oil over medium heat.
2. Add minced garlic and sauté until fragrant.
3. Add in cooked lentils and spinach.
4. Stir well and let cook for 5-7 minutes until spinach has wilted.
5. Serve as a nutritious side dish or add in some protein like grilled chicken for a complete meal.

Edamame Noodle Bowl

Ingredients:

- 1 serving soba noodles
- ½ cup steamed edamame
- 1 tablespoon sesame oil
- 1 tablespoon low-sodium soy sauce

Instructions:

1. Cook soba noodles according to package instructions.
2. In a separate pan, heat sesame oil over medium-high heat.
3. Add steamed edamame and sauté for 2-3 minutes.
4. Pour in soy sauce and continue cooking for an additional 1-2 minutes.
5. Serve noodles topped with the edamame mixture for a healthy and flavorful meal.

Snacks & Herbal Support

Sesame & Nut Energy Balls

Ingredients:

- 1 cup almond butter
- ½ cup sesame seeds
- 1 tablespoon honey
- ½ cup oats

Instructions:

1. In a mixing bowl, combine almond butter, sesame seeds, and honey.
2. Slowly add in the oats and mix until well combined.
3. Roll the mixture into small balls.
4. Store in an airtight container for up to one week.

Cucumber & Hummus Platter

Ingredients:

- 1 small cucumber, sliced
- 2 tablespoons hummus

Instructions:

1. Arrange the cucumber slices on a platter.
2. Place the hummus in a small bowl in the center of the platter.
3. Serve as a light and refreshing snack or appetizer.

Dark Chocolate & Walnut Toss

Ingredients:

- 1 ounce dark chocolate (70% or higher)
- ¼ cup walnuts

Instructions:

1. Break the dark chocolate into small pieces.
2. In a small bowl, toss together the dark chocolate and walnuts.
3. Enjoy as a satisfying and nutritious snack or dessert.

Chamomile & Lemon Tea

Ingredients:

- 1 chamomile tea bag
- 1 slice fresh lemon

Instructions:

1. Boil a cup of water in a small saucepan.
2. Add the chamomile tea bag and let it steep for 3-5 minutes.
3. Squeeze the juice from the fresh lemon slice into the tea and stir.
4. Enjoy this soothing and calming beverage as a refreshing break during your day.

Apple & Almond Butter Snack

Ingredients:

- 1 small apple, sliced
- 1 tablespoon almond butter

Instructions:

1. Slice the apple into thin wedges.
2. Spread almond butter on top of each apple slice.
3. Enjoy this healthy and delicious snack any time of day for a quick energy boost.

These recipes are easy to prepare and packed with nutrients to support your hormonal health. Enjoy experimenting with them to make meal times consistently satisfying and health-focused!

Sleep, Stress & Self-Care Essentials

When life feels overwhelming, sleep, stress management, and self-care are often the first things to fall by the wayside. Yet, these elements are foundational to your physical and mental health. Supporting your body with restorative sleep, managing stress effectively, and prioritizing self-care are powerful ways to maintain balance and resilience in your daily life. This chapter, will walk you through actionable steps for improving sleep, reducing stress, and building self-care habits that stick.

Evening Wind-Down Routines

Creating a consistent evening routine signals to your body and mind that it's time to transition from the busyness of the day to a state of rest. The goal is to reduce stimulation and promote relaxation.

- ***Set a Fixed Sleep Schedule***: Try going to bed and waking up at the same time every day—even on weekends. This consistency helps regulate your body's

internal clock, making it easier to fall asleep and wake up naturally.
- ***Dim the Lights***: About an hour before bed, reduce exposure to bright lights, especially blue light from screens. Replace screen time with softer lighting, such as lamps or candles. Consider using blue light-blocking glasses if you must use electronics.
- ***Limit Caffeine and Heavy Meals***: Avoid stimulants like caffeine in the late afternoon, and don't eat heavy meals within a couple of hours of bedtime. A light herbal tea or warm milk can be soothing alternatives.
- ***Try Calming Activities***: Swap stimulating tasks for calming ones, such as reading a book, taking a warm bath, journaling, or stretching. These promote relaxation and can help you mentally close out the day.
- ***Gratitude Practice***: Write down three things you're grateful for before bed. This simple practice helps shift your focus to positivity, easing mental tension and paving the way for restorative sleep.

Establishing an evening wind-down routine can help your body and mind transition into a restful state more easily. By incorporating small, calming habits, you set yourself up for better sleep and a more refreshed start to the day.

Natural Sleep Enhancers

Nature has a wealth of tools to help improve your sleep quality without turning to medications. Incorporate these natural sleep enhancers into your routine.

- *Magnesium*: Magnesium helps relax tense muscles and calms your nervous system. Consider magnesium-rich foods like spinach, pumpkin seeds, or dark chocolate, or take a magnesium supplement (consult your doctor first).
- *Valerian Root and Chamomile*: Herbal teas made from valerian root or chamomile can promote relaxation and improve sleep. Sip them before bedtime for a calming effect.
- *Lavender*: Aromatherapy with lavender essential oil has been shown to aid sleep. Add a few drops to your pillow or use a diffuser in your bedroom.
- *Melatonin Supplements*: For short-term sleep difficulties, melatonin supplements may help regulate your sleep cycle. Always consult a medical professional before starting any supplement.
- *White Noise or Gentle Sounds*: Use white noise machines, nature sounds, or calming music to block out distractions and create a soothing sleep environment.

Incorporating natural sleep enhancers into your routine can help you achieve better rest without relying on medications.

Experiment with these gentle, effective methods to find what works best for your body and lifestyle.

Reducing Cortisol Through Breath, Boundaries, and Balance

Chronic stress raises cortisol, wreaking havoc on your hormones, energy levels, and overall well-being. Lowering cortisol levels involves a mix of calming practices, setting boundaries, and finding a sustainable balance in your life.

- *Breathwork and Deep Breathing*: Controlled breathing techniques, such as diaphragmatic breathing, can quickly lower cortisol levels. Try this exercise: inhale deeply for four counts, hold for four counts, and exhale for six counts. Repeat this cycle for five minutes to calm your nervous system.
- *Mindfulness Practices*: Meditation, yoga, or grounding exercises help you stay rooted in the present moment, reducing the overdrive of stress responses. Even a 10-minute mindfulness session can help lower cortisol.
- *Set Boundaries*: Learning to say no and managing your time effectively are essential for reducing stress. Define clear boundaries with work, relationships, and other responsibilities to avoid becoming overwhelmed.
- *Pursue Balance*: Balance doesn't mean doing it all; it means identifying your priorities and aligning your

actions with them. Make time for activities that bring you joy, whether that's spending time with loved ones, pursuing hobbies, or simply unwinding with a good book.
- ***Physical Activity***: Gentle exercise, like walking or stretching, can reduce cortisol levels and improve your mood. Avoid intense evening workouts that may elevate stress hormones.

Sleep, stress management, and self-care are all interconnected. By investing in these areas, you're not only improving your physical health but also creating mental and emotional resilience. Small, steady changes, like creating a calming evening routine, using natural sleep aids, practicing breathwork, and prioritizing boundaries, can make a big difference over time.

Remember, self-care isn't selfish; it's essential. You can't pour from an empty cup, so make space for rest, rejuvenation, and rituals that nourish you. Start with one or two small changes from this guide today, and watch how your overall well-being improves step by step.

Beyond the Diet: Long-Term Strategies for Hormonal Wellness

Achieving hormonal wellness is not just about short-term changes. It's about creating sustainable habits that continue to support your hormones as you age. With this guide, we'll explore essential strategies to maintain balance for the long haul. From supplements to symptom tracking, learn how to keep progressing without striving for perfection.

Supplements to Consider After 40

Once you reach your 40s, hormonal shifts like perimenopause can bring new challenges. Supplements can provide targeted support to help balance hormones, boost energy, and ease symptoms. While it's always best to consult with a healthcare professional before starting any supplement, here are a few worth exploring:

- *Magnesium*: Known as nature's relaxer, magnesium supports muscle relaxation, better sleep, and stress reduction. It also helps regulate cortisol and can address symptoms like mood swings or cramps. Look for forms like magnesium glycinate for best absorption.

- ***Vitamin D***: Vitamin D supports bone health, immune function, and emotional balance. Many women are deficient, especially as they age. Sun exposure, fortified foods, and supplementation can help ensure optimal levels.
- ***Omega-3 Fatty Acids***: Omega-3s from fish oil or algae play an anti-inflammatory role and support brain, heart, and hormonal health. They may also reduce symptoms of hormonal migraines or mood swings.
- ***B Vitamins***: B-complex vitamins, particularly B6, help enhance energy, balance mood, and regulate estrogen metabolism. They're especially helpful if you're experiencing fatigue or irritability.
- ***Adaptogenic Herbs***: Herbs like ashwagandha, rhodiola, and maca work to regulate stress hormones like cortisol and promote hormonal stability. These herbs can also reduce anxiety and improve focus.
- ***Calcium and Collagen***: Supporting bone density and skin elasticity becomes more critical after 40. Calcium promotes strong bones, while collagen maintains skin and joint health.

Remember, supplements are just that—supplementary. They should complement a balanced diet and healthy lifestyle for the best results.

Tracking Symptoms and Progress

To manage hormonal wellness effectively, it's important to recognize the signs your body gives you. Tracking your symptoms and progress helps you identify patterns, see what's working, and make necessary adjustments.

Simple Tracking Methods

1. **Journaling**

    Writing things down can help you identify patterns and triggers over time. Keep track of symptoms like fatigue, mood changes, irregular cycles, hot flashes, or sleep issues, and jot down when they occur.

    Also, include notes about lifestyle factors such as your diet, exercise routine, stress levels, and sleep quality. This can provide valuable insights when discussing your health with a professional.

2. **Apps**

    Hormone health tracking apps are great tools for staying consistent with your monitoring. These apps allow you to log your cycles, moods, and physical symptoms quickly and easily, even on busy days. Some apps also offer detailed charts, reminders, or tips tailored to your hormonal health. Choose one that best fits your needs and the features most relevant to your goals.

3. **Lab Testing**

   Regular bloodwork is an important step in understanding your hormonal health. Testing key hormones like estrogen, progesterone, cortisol, and thyroid levels can reveal imbalances that may be affecting your well-being.

   Partnering with a healthcare provider to interpret these results ensures you can take the right steps toward improving your health. You might also explore additional testing options depending on your symptoms, such as checking for vitamin deficiencies or adrenal function.

What to Look For

- *Improved Sleep*: Less tossing and turning, deeper rest.
- *Consistent Energy*: Feeling less drained throughout the day.
- *Mood Stability*: Fewer swings in mood or irritability.
- *Reduced Symptoms*: A noticeable decline in hot flashes, bloating, or painful cycles.

By tracking your progress, you empower yourself to make informed decisions that continually improve your hormonal health.

Staying Consistent Without Being Perfect

Perfection is overrated. Hormonal wellness doesn't demand flawless eating habits, stress-free days, or a spotless supplement schedule. Life happens, and the goal is progress, not perfection. Here's how to stay consistent without falling into an all-or-nothing mindset:

1. **Adopt the 80/20 Rule**

    Strive to follow your hormone-friendly habits 80% of the time while leaving room for flexibility in the remaining 20%. This means focusing on nutrient-rich meals, regular exercise, and stress management most of the time, but also recognizing that life isn't perfect.

    One indulgent dessert, an unplanned meal out, or a skipped workout won't derail your progress. In fact, allowing yourself occasional treats or breaks can make your plan more sustainable and enjoyable in the long run, helping you stay consistent without feeling deprived or restricted. Balance is key!

2. **Build Small, Sustainable Habits**

    Big changes can feel overwhelming, so focus on one habit at a time. For instance:

    - Start your mornings with a hormone-friendly smoothie three times a week.

- Incorporate magnesium-rich snacks like almonds or dark chocolate into your routine.
- Add a 10-minute mindfulness session to your evening wind-down.

Small but consistent habits can lead to significant changes over time.

3. Forgive Setbacks

We all have busy weeks that throw us off track, whether it's a demanding work schedule, unexpected travel, or unplanned stressors. It's completely normal to face challenges that disrupt your routine. If you hit a bump in the road, don't stress or dwell on it.

Instead, take a moment to reflect on what happened, acknowledge it without judgment, and remind yourself that setbacks are part of the process. When you're ready, pick up where you left off and keep moving forward. Progress isn't about perfection—it's about perseverance.

4. Focus on How You Feel

Instead of striving for a specific number on the scale or sticking to a rigid diet plan, pay attention to how you feel as a measure of your progress. This could mean noticing that you have more energy throughout the day, experiencing fewer mood swings, feeling less stressed, or enjoying better quality sleep.

By tuning into these internal changes, you can build a healthier relationship with your goals and create a positive mindset that celebrates sustainable improvements, rather than external metrics alone.

5. **Create a Support Network**

Share your health goals with a friend, partner, or support group. Having someone to check in with can keep you accountable and motivated. You're not alone, and building a community around these goals adds encouragement and fun.

Hormonal wellness is a marathon, not a sprint. Your body evolves with time, so allow your efforts to evolve as well. Periodically revisit this guide, adjust strategies as needed, and stay flexible. It's these small, consistent, and mindful changes that will help you maintain hormonal balance for the long haul.

Conclusion

Balancing estrogen levels isn't just about managing hormones; it's about reclaiming control over your health and vitality. For women over 40, maintaining healthy estrogen levels can influence everything from energy and mood to sleep and overall well-being. While your body naturally goes through changes during this phase of life, you have the power to support this transition and thrive in the process. Small, intentional choices can pave the way for a vibrant, balanced life.

Throughout this guide, we've explored the impact of diet, lifestyle, and environmental factors on estrogen health. Now it's time to put those insights into action. Begin with the foundation of nutrition. Prioritize fiber-rich vegetables, whole grains, healthy fats, and lean proteins to support hormone regulation and promote gut health. Incorporate phytoestrogen-rich foods like flaxseeds and soy in moderation, while limiting processed foods, refined sugars, and unhealthy fats that can disrupt hormonal balance. Hydration plays a vital role as well, so drink plenty of filtered water each day to support detoxification and cellular health.

Your lifestyle choices matter just as much as the food on your plate. Consistent, moderate exercise helps keep stress hormones in check, maintains a healthy weight, and supports overall hormonal harmony. But balance is key! Over-exercising or completely skipping movement can strain your system. Find an activity you enjoy, whether it's walking, yoga, cycling, or dancing, and make it a regular part of your routine.

Stress management is another crucial piece of the puzzle. Chronic stress can wreak havoc on your hormones, so adopting stress-relief practices like mindfulness, meditation, or deep breathing is essential. Don't forget to make sleep a priority, too. Aim for seven to nine hours of high-quality rest each night to allow your body time to repair and reset. Remember, sleep is not a luxury; it's a necessity, particularly when it comes to hormone health.

We also discussed the role of environmental toxins in disrupting your hormones. You can minimize your exposure by choosing BPA-free containers, switching to natural or eco-friendly cleaning products, and avoiding personal care products with parabens, phthalates, and synthetic fragrances. Even small swaps, like filtered water and non-toxic cookware, can reduce your toxin burden over time, allowing your body to function at its best.

Above all, remember that balance doesn't require perfection. It's about making informed decisions that align with your health goals. Start with just one or two changes today and build on them as you go. Whether it's swapping plastic containers for glass, adding more greens to your meals, or carving out time for self-care, every step counts toward creating a healthier, happier future.

By taking ownership of your diet, environment, and daily habits, you're giving your body the tools to function optimally. This isn't just about managing symptoms or getting through menopause; it's about living a life filled with energy, confidence, and purpose.

Thank you for taking the time to complete this guide. Your health is worth the investment, and we're thrilled you've taken this meaningful step toward a balanced, vibrant life. Here's to your health, your happiness, and your empowered future!

FAQs

Why is balancing estrogen levels important for women over 40?

Balancing estrogen levels supports a range of health factors, including mood, energy, sleep, and overall well-being. During perimenopause and menopause, estrogen levels can fluctuate, leading to symptoms like fatigue, weight gain, and mood swings. Taking steps to balance estrogen helps ease these transitions and promotes vitality.

What are phytoestrogens, and should I include them in my diet?

Phytoestrogens are plant-based compounds that mimic estrogen in the body. Foods like flaxseeds, soy, and lentils contain them. Including moderate amounts of these in your diet may help balance estrogen levels, but overconsumption may not be beneficial. It's best to focus on variety and moderation.

What foods should I avoid to improve hormone health?

Limit processed foods, refined sugars, trans fats, and high-intake of alcohol. These can disrupt hormone balance and contribute to inflammation or weight gain. Instead, prioritize whole, nutrient-dense foods that support overall health and hormonal function.

Can reducing exposure to toxins really make a difference in hormone balance?

Yes! Many environmental toxins act as endocrine disruptors, which can interfere with your hormonal system and mimic estrogen. By using BPA-free containers, natural cleaning products, and non-toxic personal care items, you reduce this impact and support your body's natural hormone regulation.

How does exercise impact estrogen levels?

Regular, moderate exercise helps maintain a healthy weight, manage stress hormones, support better sleep, and improve overall well-being, all of which contribute to balancing estrogen. However, over-exercising can lead to hormonal imbalances, so finding a sustainable routine is key.

How can I better manage stress to balance hormones?

Stress has a significant effect on your hormones. Practices like mindfulness, meditation, deep breathing, or yoga can lower cortisol levels and improve hormonal harmony. Carving out time for relaxation and activities you enjoy is just as important as other health measures.

Can small changes really make a difference, or do I need a complete lifestyle overhaul?

Small, steady changes can absolutely make a difference! Switching to better food choices, reducing toxin exposure, or setting time aside for sleep and stress management are manageable steps that lead to significant long-term benefits. Build on these gradually to create sustainable habits.

References and Helpful Links

Rd, J. K. M. (2020, November 30). How your diet can affect estrogen levels. Healthline.
https://www.healthline.com/nutrition/foods-to-lower-estrogen

Lord, D. (2023, October 24). Symptoms of hormonal changes at 40. Nava Health.
https://navacenter.com/symptoms-of-hormonal-changes-at-40/

Johnson, E. (2024, February 24). Lifestyle factors and hormone levels. BodyLogicMD.
https://www.bodylogicmd.com/blog/lifestyle-factors-and-hormone-levels/

NEXtCARE. (2025, February 5). Hormone-Happy Food: 6 recipes to support healthy harmony - NextCare. Nextcare.
https://www.nextcarehealth.com/news/hormone-happy-food-6-recipes-to-support-healthy-harmony/

Cpt, K. D. M. R. (2024b, January 29). 11 natural ways to lower your cortisol levels. Healthline.
https://www.healthline.com/nutrition/ways-to-lower-cortisol

Breathing exercises for beating stress and creating calm: a guide for teachers and education staff. (n.d.). https://www.educationsupport.org.uk/resources/for-individuals/guides/breathing-exercises-for-beating-stress-and-creating-calm/

Robinson, L., & Smith, M., MA. (2025, March 13). Stress Management: Techniques to Deal with Stress. HelpGuide.org. https://www.helpguide.org/mental-health/stress/stress-management

www.ingramcontent.com/pod-product-compliance
Lightning Source LLC
LaVergne TN
LVHW012030060526
838201LV00061B/4533